MW00465612

How to Start a Nail Salon Business

ISBN-13: 978-1477690710

ISBN-10: 1477690719

Copyright Notice

HOW TO START A
NAIL SALON BUSINESS

Essential Start-Up Tips to Boost Your Nail Salon Business Success

Una Algrier

I dedicate this book to every person – be they woman (or man) whose lives have been touched by the joy, excitement and sheer fun of getting their nails done...

Contents

Nail Salon Business
An Introduction

When you look at a nail technician practicing their craft, the work may seem easy, but it actually requires a great deal of skill.

The good thing is that once you've started a career as a nail technician or nail artist, it can be very profitable and a lot of fun.

Having fun can be very important in a field where hard work and dedication are needed in order to achieve expertise and success.

As a nail technician, you'll have the option of working in a nail salon or starting a salon of your own.

And because the nail salon business has become a fast-growing industry, many nail technicians have chosen to open their own business.

Local

A lot of people choose to set up nail salons in their locality or as near their neighbourhoods as possible. This is because people are busy these days and prefer to go to salon that is near to their home.

And nail art has become so popular that men and women alike are now taking courses in nail maintenance and beautification. Many of those who complete such courses then find gainful and fun employment at nail salons.

If you want to become an expert nail technician, however, you'll have to go through a lengthy process of developing and enhancing your craft. And when you feel ready to start your own nail salon business, then it's advisable for you to take classes in running the business as well to complement your knowledge in nail art.

After all, there's a significant difference between simply practicing your craft and running a successful business venture.

If you truly have a passion for making other people beautiful, then starting your own nail salon business may indeed be an excellent idea. Other than allowing you to serve other people, a nail salon can also be a very profitable business.

It takes special skills to become a professional nail technician. If you've already received the necessary training and have worked as a nail technician for some time, then you may be thinking of starting your own nail salon business.

If that's the case, then now is the perfect time to take the plunge.

The Basics

Nail salons can range from small kiosks that offer quick and limited services to elaborate nail spas that provide you with luxurious treatments.

Although there are already hundreds of nail salons everywhere and it seems that there's no longer any room for one more, there are still ways for you to start your own nail salon and make a success out of it.

The key is in setting yourself apart from the competition and making your business stand out. The best thing is that it's easy enough to get started as long as you have the necessary knowledge and skills.

Here are some straightforward guidelines you can follow:

1. Find out what the requirements are as regards permits and licenses for your business.

   Be sure to research the licensing requirements both for a nail salon business and a professional nail technician.

   As the business owner, you may not be required to secure a professional nail tech license, but your employees surely will.

   It's important that you comply with all legal requirements to make sure you don't run into any problems down the line.

   Take note that the health board in most localities require nail technicians to be duly licensed and state certified, so make sure you have all the necessary permits and licenses to practice.

Otherwise, make sure you have a duly-licensed nail technician in your employ. Of course, you'll also need a business license and any other permit or license required by your locality. Take care of all these requirements so you won't run into any legal problems in the future.

2. Consider the type of services you'll be offering in your nail salon.

   Manicures, pedicures, gel nails, acrylic nails, fibreglass nails, and airbrushing are among the most basic services offered by most nail salons.

   Once you've decided on your services, you should set the price for each type of service you'll be offering. This can be accomplished by identifying the equipment and supplies needed and then finding out how much it'll cost you to obtain them.

   You should also determine how much space you'll need to be able to offer all of the services you want to offer.

   This will help you find the right location for your salon.

3. Once you've found the right location, decide if you're going to buy the property or just lease it.

Negotiate favourable selling or leasing terms with the property owner.

Before you close the sale or sign the lease, make sure the property has adequate ventilation, since some of the chemicals used in nail art can be harmful when inhaled in large amounts.

You should also ensure that the plumbing is in good working order.

You'd also do well to discuss possible renovations if you're leasing the property.

4. Hire the necessary employees and ensure they get proper training.

   It may be a good idea to draft a code of ethics and some house rules, so that each of your employees clearly understands how you expect things to run in your nail salon.

5. Advertise your nail salon business.

   Put up an attractive signage outside your salon and design attractive posters advertising the services you offer as well.

   Display these posters on your front windows and on the reception counter.

Have business cards and flyers printed as well and then distribute them outside grocery stores, malls, and even college campuses.

You may also want to consider having a grand opening promotion where you offer discounts to the first 50 customers or so.

6. Prepare a business plan.

   This document serves two very important purposes.

   First, it can serve as your guide to make sure you're taking all the necessary steps in starting and operating your nail salon, thus helping ensure the success of your business.

   Second, it can be a very important tool in securing financing for your new business. Your business plan should contain the details of how you plan to start your business, what direction you intend for it to take, and how you intend to get there.

   Estimates of start-up cost, projections of future income, and a solid marketing plan should all be part of your business plan.

7. Secure the necessary financing to set-up your nail salon business.

This is when you can put your business plan to good use.

Take note that banks and other lending institutions are more likely to entertain the idea of providing you with the necessary amount to start your business if you have a solid business plan on hand.

The business plan assures them of two things.

First, that you know exactly what you're getting into, and second, that you have a truly viable way of paying them back.

8. Find the right location for your nail salon.

   Sometimes it's a good idea to set up shop near another nail salon, but sometimes it's not.

   You'll have to learn how to make the distinction.

   Better yet, identify your target market first and then set up shop at a location that your target market frequents.

   For example, if you want to cater to young professionals wanting to look good whether at work or on special occasions, then it may be a good idea to set up your salon near office buildings or apartment complexes where your target customers are likely to be found.

9. Decide how big you want your salon to be for starters.

   This will determine how many people you'll need to hire.

   For example, if you decide to have a nail salon that can cater to just five customers at once, then you'll probably need just two nail technicians besides yourself, a couple of assistants, and someone to man the counter.

   For running a bigger salon, you'll naturally need more staff as well.

10. Get some background in business management if you don't have one already.

    This is important if you want to keep on top of things in any type of business.

    Above all, make sure your services are always of top quality.

    More than anything else, excellent service is what keeps customers coming back. With the right approach, you can surely look forward to attaining business success in no time at all.

    So now we have covered the overview let's get down to specifics.

Naming Your
Nail Salon Business

Choosing a company name can be the most fun part of starting a company. It can also be one of the most important.

After all, having the right nail salon business name can be a very effective advertising tool.

Among other things, it can give prospective customers a general idea of what your company does and what you have to offer.

In the same way, choosing the wrong name is likely to drive would-be customers away.

Here are a couple of things to remember when choosing a nail salon business name:

Keep it short and memorable

Needless to say, a short company name is much easier to remember than a lengthy one.

Choosing a short name doesn't just involve using less words, but also words with less syllables.

But, aside from being short, your nail salon business name also has to be catchy so as to promote better name recall.

You are your name

This means your company name should reflect the company's personality. It should give people a general idea of what services you provide or what benefits they can get from patronizing your nail salon business.

You need to have an image which you want your nail salon business to project and the name you choose must fit that image.

More importantly, you have to choose a name your target customers can easily connect with.
Now, you know the basics of choosing a company name and you realize how important a name is to your business.

However, you shouldn't take the process of choosing a name too seriously.

While the company name does have to reflect its personality, it doesn't really have to define your company completely.

Take note that venturing into other related businesses is a normal part of any company's growth, so there is a real possibility that you may have to change your nail salon business name from time to time.

Again, the name of your nail salon business is important, but you shouldn't get hung up on the process of choosing it.

As long as you make sure that it's memorable, it tells people what your nail salon business is about, and you're proud of it, then you're good to go.

Communication for Success

You should realise, though, that more than these things, you'll need to be able to develop a solid relationship with your clients.

Remember that if clients don't feel comfortable with you and your staff, then they aren't likely to return and will probably take their business somewhere else. That's definitely something you don't want to happen. What you need to aim for is to keep your customers coming back and possibly even bring family and friends with them.

In a nail salon business, as with many other kinds of business, first impressions often have a significant impact on how the business fares in the long term.

Therefore, you should strive to give your clients a positive first impression of your nail salon. You or a member of your staff should always be ready to greet a client as soon as he or she enters the door. And while they're waiting in your reception area, clients should be directed to magazines and other reading materials. They should also be asked if there's anything else they need.

It's also a huge advantage if you hire a receptionist who doesn't just sit silently at the front desk, but is willing to strike up a conversation with your clients while they wait to be served.

Communication is indeed the key to winning repeat customers. And with effective communication, these repeat customers will soon seem more like friends. In any kind of business, excellent customer service is highly valuable and one of the key aspects of excellent service is effective communication. This is why you always need to find fresh ways of keeping the communication lines open between you and your clients.

Here are some of the most significant benefits you can enjoy as a result of effective communication:

1. The ability to communicate well with others makes an individual naturally cheerful. This positivity, in turn, will help you create a happy atmosphere in your nail salon. This is something your clients will surely appreciate and may even be one of the main reasons why they would decide to come back and recommend your business to others.

2. If you're able to build a positive atmosphere in your nail salon, then you're bound to create a buzz within salon-going individuals. This will help you build a reputation for excellent service that's sure to earn you a steady stream of clients.

3. As a result of effective communication, you should be able to create a strong bond with your loyal clients. Good communication, after all, helps build friendships as well as healthy professional relationships.

4. With good communication, you're also able to create a relaxed atmosphere in your nail salon both for your clients and your staff. This is very important because when your employees are stressed, then they're likely to take their frustration out on your clients. But, if they work in a relaxed atmosphere, then they're likely to be more amiable to clients.

5. The ability to communicate well naturally helps you understand your clients better. By understanding them better, you also understand their needs better and will be better able to keep them satisfied.

Drawing Up a Business Plan

Developing a new nail salon business naturally requires a good foundation, and building such a foundation begins with having a sound business plan.

Remember that the business plan is an essential part of documenting a start-up business' financial goals, business objectives, and marketing plans.

Implementation of all your nail salon business ideas can only successfully begin once you've completed your business plan.

Your Business Plan: Choosing the Right Format

You probably already know that a business plan ranks among the most vital components of starting your business and ensuring its success. But, how exactly do you make a good business plan? Well, there are several variations and templates you can choose from. What's important is for you to choose the one that's best suited to the kind of enterprise you'll be running and to the purpose for which you're making the plan in the first place.

Here are some of the things you need to take into consideration:

1. Your Target Audience

There are two types of business plan.

a. There are business plans intended for an internal audience and these plans are usually part of your business growth strategy; they're also usually referred to as strategic plans.

b. There are also plans meant for external audiences and the purpose of these plans is usually to attract financing, suppliers, or talent for your business.

If the purpose of your business plan is primarily to get funding, then the document will typically be in condensed form, or a sort of summary of a more comprehensive business plan.

Such a version is generally known as a *funding proposal* or a *business opportunity document* and it's usually followed by the larger plan.

A business plan can indeed be a very useful document, so it's important to clearly define the audience for which it is intended.

2. What Goes Into the Plan?

Remember that a business plan needs to be comprehensive and that it's essentially created to put into writing what you envision for your business venture.

Your business plan should contain:

- An executive summary,
- The background and history of your company,
- A clear description of your nail salon business concept,
- Your marketing analysis and development plan,
- Your operations and production assessment,
- Your financial assessments and projections,
- Your human resources management assessment and plan,
- Your business implementation plan,

- An identification of resources,
- The proposed investor deal structures wherever appropriate,
- A survival strategy that describes potential risks and mitigation measures,
- Your nail salon business growth strategy,
- Your exit strategy,
- Appendices.

If that seems daunting, don't worry. Some of the components of your business plan may be longer than others and some of them are optional, depending on your target audience, the format you choose to adopt, and the purpose of your plan.

What's important is for your intended reader to clearly grasp the value proposition, understand why your nail salon business is expected to succeed, and how that success will be achieved.

If you're pitching the plan to potential investors, (or most probably the bank) then they should quickly understand your proposed deal structure and the possible returns.

3. What Length To Make Your Plan

The average business plan typically consists of 20 pages, though there are some that contain a hundred pages or more. The length of your plan will depend largely on its purpose and your target audience.
If the primary purpose of your business plan is to attract investors, then you can expect it to contain more details and therefore be lengthier than a plan that's primarily for communicating your business growth strategy.

In the same way, the business plan for a venture with a relatively simple concept should be a lot more concise than one that's made for a highly complicated enterprise.

4. Should You Use a Template or Pay a Consultant?

Many people are also confused as to whether they should hire a consultant to help them write their business plan or simply use a template for guidance. Well, it can be quite tempting to use a template or get someone else to make the plan for you. However, it's still best if you write the plan yourself even if you do decide to get some guidance from a consultant. After all, who knows your business better than you?

A solid business plan is perhaps the easiest way for you to communicate your nail salon business ideas to your target audience as well as to help you prevent problems and identify business growth strategies.

It can also be your most valuable tool when you're in search of funding for your nail salon business.

Remember, though, that instead of treating it as a blueprint or a strict manual which you should implement to the letter, the plan should be seen as more of a guide in operating your nail salon business. TIP: Even if you don't have an immediate audience for your plan, the document and even the process itself will definitely prove to be of value to your business in the long run.

Preparing a solid business plan for all the right reasons can indeed increase your chances of attaining success in your nail salon business.

How to Write the Executive Summary

The executive summary generally serves as the introduction to your formal and comprehensive business plan.

You could even say that this is Part 1 of your business plan.

It contains a summary of your nail salon business proposition, present business status, financial projections, and the key elements for success.

Although it's often tempting to just rush through this component of your business plan, always remember that an executive summary is likely to be the very first thing your target investors or banking officials will read in the document. It basically tells the reader the status of the company currently, and where it's expected to go. Many people aren't likely to read the remainder of the plan if the executive summary doesn't catch their interest, so it's really very important to do this right.

The importance of the executive summary lies in the fact that it tells your reader exactly why you believe your nail salon business will be a success.

Brevity is the key to a solid executive summary, which generally ranges from half a page to a maximum of two pages. Writing anything longer puts you at risk of losing the reader's attention and appearing unfocused. If you can keep the summary under one page without sacrificing quality, then do so.

Note: Although it serves as the introduction, it's best to write the executive summary after you've completed your business plan. After all, it is basically a shorter version of your plan.

To keep the summary consistent with the plan itself, it should have the following components:

1. Your Mission Statement

Your business plan's executive summary is be the best place for you to express your mission statement. Make sure that statement is concise and explains in as few words as possible the existence of your nail salon business, its goals, and how you plan to achieve those goals.

In short, it should explain your nail salon business thrust to the reader. Remember to keep your mission statement focused and direct, leaving no room for confusion as regards what your nail salon business venture is all about.

2. What's Your Business Concept?

In describing your nail salon business concept, you'll need to offer some details about the kind of nail salon business you'll be running, who your target customers are, and what your competitive advantages are.

You may point out that you're filling a void you've identified in the market, offering better prices for comparable services in the industry, or offering a better service than what's currently available.

3. A Little Background

You may also want to give your reader an idea of when your venture began, who the founders are and what functions they perform, how many employees you have (or plan to hire), and where the nail salon business is located and if there are any subsidiaries or branches. A description of your offices and facilities as well as the services your offer would also be a good idea.

4. Your Nail Salon Business Status and Financial Outlook

You'll also need to give a short description of the current status of your nail salon business. Explain if your business is still in the conceptualization stage, if you've already started setting it up, or if it's already fully operational and you're simply planning to expand.

You should also mention your expected costs and your financial projections for both the short term and the long term.

This will give potential investors an idea of how much capital you need and if your business venture matches the kind of opportunity they're currently looking for. If you already have existing investors, then you'd do well to provide some information on them as well.

5. Key Factors for Success

The reader of your business plan will also appreciate getting a preview of the key factors for nail salon business success. These factors depend on your situation, of course, but it generally includes technology patents, strategic partnerships, market factors and economic trends.

If your nail salon business is already fully operational and you've had some successful projects worth noting (you may have been the first to offer a certain service in the industry), then you should include that as well.

Finally...

All in all, your business plan's executive summary should provide its reader with a quick but insightful glimpse into the plan itself.

It's advisable to highlight everything except the mission statement in bulleted lists. Include all of the important points without revealing too much, since each section is discussed in detail within the plan itself, anyway.

More importantly, make sure the summary sells the proposal on its own as much as possible, just in case reader doesn't read your plan. It does happen!

Note: It's also a good idea to draw up a table of contents right after the executive summary so the reader will know where he can find each section in the plan itself.

If you're still in the process of setting up your nail salon business, then you likely won't have much to write as regards to some of the areas listed above. In that case, focus on your own experience and expertise in the field, and the circumstances that led to your nail salon business concept.

Tell your target readers how you plan to set your nail salon business apart from the competition and convince them that there's indeed a need for your business within your target niche or industry.

Company History

After the executive summary, your business plan should contain a section covering your business background or company history. The length of this portion and how it's told will depend largely on how far along your nail salon business is in terms of operations and development.

Naturally, the business history of a venture that's just starting is totally different from one that's been operating for some time. It should be about one page long, though it's understandable for a start-up company's history to cover less than an entire page.

What to Include

In this section, you should be able to illustrate how the various elements of your nail salon business venture fit together and form one successful enterprise.

You should also include some background information on the nature of the nail salon business itself and identify the factors that are expected to facilitate its success.

Furthermore, don't forget to mention the specific market needs you're planning to satisfy and the ways and methods in which you expect to satisfy these needs. If possible, you should also identify the specific individuals or groups of people whom you believe have those needs.

An example of a specific market could be:

Women aged 18 to 30 with an income of $80,000 within 50 miles of your location.

How It All Started

Among the things you should include in the company history portion of your business plan is the origin of your nail salon business concept.

This explains how you first came upon the idea for your nail salon business and why you decided to pursue that idea. You should also indicate the progress you've made so far as regards operating and growing your business venture. If you're still in the process of starting your business, then say so.

NOTE: It's also a good idea to mention the problems you've encountered along the way and how you handled each of them. Potential investors and business partners will surely appreciate knowing that they're dealing with someone who's not afraid to deal with challenges from time to time.

Projected Short-Term Growth

You would also do well to include your short-term business growth plans in this section, so the reader will know that you've thought about your venture carefully and that you have concrete plans for its growth.

NOTE: If you're just starting a new nail salon business, then you may want to include a bit of personal history along with your background.

Among the things you can include are your educational history, technical skills, areas of expertise, relevant professional club memberships, and other nail salon businesses you may have started or companies you worked for.

TIP: You may even want to share your areas of inexperience or weaknesses and how you intend to compensate for these areas. Your target investors would definitely appreciate knowing that you're aware of the things you need to improve on and are making concrete efforts at improving them.

Finally...

In summary, the company history section of your business plan should provide an interested reader with a much better idea of how your nail salon business came to be and who you are as a businessperson.

Again, the key is to keep this section concise and avoiding unwanted information.

Organization and Management

This section of your plan includes the following:

- Your company's organizational structure

- The profiles of your management team

- Details about company ownership

- The board of director's qualifications

It's important for you to answer the question of who does what when you prepare this section. Explain what each person's background and qualifications are. Tell your reader exactly why you've brought or are bringing these people into your organization and management team. What exactly are they responsible and accountable for?

NOTE: You may think this section of the plan is unnecessary if you're setting up a small venture with less than five people on your team, but anybody reading your business plan needs to know who's in charge.

Therefore, you should still provide a description of every department or division, along with their functions, regardless of the size of your company.

If there's an advisory board for your business, then you should also identify who's on it and how you plan to keep each member on the board.

- What salary and benefits do you plan to provide for members of your team?

- Will you be offering incentives? If so, what are they?

- How do you plan to handle promotions?

In this section of your business plan, you need to reassure your audience that the people on your team aren't going to be just names on your company letterhead.

What's Your Structure?

One very simple yet effective way of presenting your organizational structure is by creating an organizational chart and then providing a narrative description of the chart.

By doing this, you don't leave anything to chance, you're making sure the functions and responsibilities of each team member has been carefully thought out, and you've ensured that someone's in charge of each and every function in your nail salon business. Therefore, no function is taken for granted and there'll be no overlapping of responsibilities.

TIP: Remember that this kind of assurance is very important to your reader, especially if that reader is a potential investor.

Management Profiles

Ask any business expert and he'll probably tell you that among the most significant success factors in any business is the track record and ability of the management team.

This is why it's important for you to provide your reader with a background of the key members of the management team.

Specifically, you'd do well to provide resumes that indicate the name, position and the corresponding functions, primary responsibilities and level of authority, educational background, skills and experience, number of years on your team (unless it's a start-up company), compensation level and basis, previous employment and track record, industry recognitions received, and community involvement. TIP: When you indicate the track record of your team, be sure to quantify their achievements.

For example, instead of saying:

"Extensive experience in managing a sales department"

you could say:

"Successfully managed a sales department of ten people for 15 years."

It's also a good idea to highlight how the key members of the management team complement your own experience and expertise.

If you're starting a new nail salon business, then show your reader how the unique experiences of each member of your team can contribute to your business venture's overall success.

Company Ownership

Aside from the organizational structure, this section of the plan should also describe the legal structure and provide important ownership information regarding your nail salon business.

- Has the business been incorporated? If so, then is it an S or a C corporation?

- Is your business a partnership?

- If so, then is it a limited or general partnership?

- Or are you the sole proprietor of your nail salon business?

The most important pieces of information you should include in this section are the owner/s' names, ownership percentage, form of ownership, degree of involvement of each owner within the business, common stock, and outstanding equity equivalents.

Board Qualifications

Take note that there's a huge advantage to setting up an unpaid board of advisors for your company, as it can provide you with the kind of expertise the company is otherwise unable to afford.

Simply by enlisting the help of some successful businessmen who are popular in the industry and including them in your advisory board, you'll definitely go far in enhancing the credibility of your company and encouraging a perception of expertise.

If the company has a board of directors, then you need to provide the names of the board members, their respective positions in the BOD, their background, the extent of their involvement with the nail salon business, and their expected contribution to its success.

Market Analysis

You may be a hundred percent confident about the quality of the service your nail salon business has to offer, but unless you're able to connect with your target customers, quality won't do you much good. You'll have to get your service into your customers' hands, so to speak, to get the necessary sales. And that's why you need market analysis. This section of your business plan should be used to illustrate your knowledge of the industry. You may also use it to present highlights and conclusions from the marketing research data you've collected.

For your analysis to be reliable, you need to study the three Cs of marketing:

1. Company

2. Customer

3. Competition

Of course, it's understandable that you should be aware of your company's strengths and weaknesses, but you should also know the same things about your competitors so you'll get a better idea of how to deal with them.

More importantly, you need to know who your customers are and what their needs and wants really are.

When you prepare the company analysis component of this section, you'll need to describe the primary industry to which your business belongs, the industry's current size and historic growth rate, the industry's characteristics and trends, and the industry's major customer groups.

All these will put into perspective the description you'll provide of the company you've established or are planning to establish.

Who Are Your Target Customers?

In choosing and defining your target customers, make sure that you narrow it down to a size that you're sure you can manage.

Many business owners make the mistake of trying to provide everything to everybody at once. Slow and sure is often a better philosophy where your business is concerned.

This section of your plan should include information that identifies the unique characteristics of your target customers including:

- Their needs

- The extent to which these needs are being met

- Demographics.

It's also a good idea to identify your target market's geographic location, who among them makes the major decisions, and any market trends that may affect your business. The size of your target market should also be indicated in this section, along with your expected market share gains and the reason for these expected gains. You should also indicate your pricing schedule as well as your gross margin targets and whatever discount structures you may be planning. You'd also do well to identify what resources you plan to use to get information as regards your target market, the media you'll be using to reach the market, your target market's purchasing cycle, and the socio-economic trends likely to affect your target market.

If all this sounds complicated don't worry, just break down each section and do it one at a time.

Your Competition

Of all the Cs you need to study, your competition may be the toughest, especially if you're new to the industry. The first thing you need to do is study your direct competitors.

If you're planning to operate a nail salon business in your district, then you're likely to get direct competition from the likes of the larger multi-national nail salon businesses. So it pays to examine all the possible options on how you can set your nail salon business apart.

It's important for you to identify your direct competitors according to product or service line and market segment.

You should then assess their weaknesses and strengths, determine the level of importance of your own target market to your competitors, and identify the barriers that may pose a challenge as you enter your target niche.

This may include high investment costs, changing technology, existing patents or trademarks, customer resistance, and a difficulty in finding quality personnel.

You'd also do well to determine the market share of each key competitor and then provide an estimate of the time it'll take for new competitors to enter the niche. Aside from looking for ways to set yourself apart from the competition, you'll also want to see how your business fits into the marketplace itself.

In doing so, you'll have to consider the strengths and weaknesses of your competitors, the possibility of competitors leaving the marketplace and new ones entering it, the services your competitors are relying on for a majority of their revenue, and effective ways of overcoming possible threats from substitute services.

Developing Your Marketing Strategy

Once all three Cs have been addressed, you should be ready to start developing your marketing program. This basically involves an analysis of what's known as the "four Ps."

They are:

1. Product

2. Place

3. Price

4. Promotion

Product, of course, refers to what you plan to sell (in this case your nail salon service) Place refers to where you plan to sell it (office, online, or both).

Price refers to the amount you'll charge for each service you'll be offering.
And Promotion refers to the incentives and other promotional strategies you plan to use in order to get your target market to try your services.

To put it simply, a marketing strategy is your way of drawing in customers, which is indeed very important since customers are essentially the lifeblood of any business venture.

There isn't a single way of approaching a marketing strategy.

What's important is for your strategy to be uniquely applicable to your nail salon business and part of a continuing evaluation process that aims to facilitate business growth and success.

In conducting a "four Ps" analysis, you'll likely conduct some market tests and you'd do well to include the results of these tests in this section of your business plan. All other details of the tests may be attached as an appendix.

The information you provide in this section may include the number of customers who participated in the tests, demonstrations or any information provided to the participating customers, the degree of importance of satisfying the needs of your target market, and the percentage of participants who expressed desire to take advantage of your products and/or services.

After creating your marketing strategy, you'll also need to draw up a sales strategy, which outlines the methods you'll be using to actually sell the services you plan to offer.

There are two very important elements of a good sales strategy.

- The first is your sales force strategy, which determines if you'll be employing internal sales personnel or independent representatives. You should also identify the number of people you plan to recruit for your company's sales force as well as the recruitment and training strategies you'll be using. You'd also do well to present the compensation packages you've lined up for your sales personnel.

- The second element of a sales strategy is a description of the sales activities you've lined up for the company.

A sales strategy is made more manageable when broken down into activities.

For example, you could start with identifying prospective customers and then prioritizing your prospects according to those who have the highest potential of buying your products.

From this outline of activities, you can easily determine the number of prospects you may have to get to make a sale and the average amount you'll likely earn from each sale. You'll also need to draw up a solid market development plan in order to make your market analysis work to your advantage. While the information in your development plan is likely to come into play only when your company has been established and operational for at least a few years, potential investors will surely appreciate the fact that you've already envisioned your company's growth and evolution.

Among other things, your development plan should provide answers to the following questions:

> Is the market for the services you offer currently growing?

> Are you planning to offer line extensions or new services within your first few years of operations?

> Does the market development plan you've crafted offer ways of increasing the overall demand for your services within the industry?

> Are there alternative ways of making your company more competitive?

Remember that the market analysis is a vital part of your business plan and it's likely to take up a large part of the plan itself.

This is why it's necessary to conduct a thorough research on the competition and on the market you're planning to enter.

Note

You may have the best service in the market, but without an organized and well-crafted market analysis and development plan, you still won't be able to guarantee success.

You market analysis helps you identify a clear roadmap of how to bring your services to your target customers.

Financial Projections

Making financial projections for a start-up nail salon business can be described as both science and art. Investors may want to see you spell out financial forecasts in cold, hard numbers, but it's not really that easy to predict the financial performance of your nail salon business several years from now, especially if you're still in the process of raising capital.

Simply put, this is the part where you formally request funding from potential investors and you do that by illustrating how much funding you need for start-up as well as within the first five years of operations.

If you already have an existing business and are looking towards expansion, then you may reflect the funding requirements for the expansion itself.

Potential investors are also sure to appreciate some historical data as regards the financial performance of your company, particularly within the last three years or so, depending on how long you've been in business. If you have any collateral that can possibly be used to secure a loan, then that's worth noting as well.

Difficulty aside, financial projections are requirements for a solid business plan and you'll really have to deal with them if you truly want to catch your prospective investors' attention. Regardless of whether your business is a start-up or a growing venture, you'll still need to provide historical and/or projected financial data.

Here are a few useful tips:

1. **Don't let spreadsheets intimidate you**

All financial projections necessarily start with spreadsheet software, with Microsoft Excel being the most commonly used; chances are great you already have the software on your computer.
Other than this, there are also some special software packages that can help you with financial projections. These packages often provide flexibility, which allows you to weigh alternate scenarios or change assumptions quickly whenever necessary.

2. **Create short-term projections as well as medium-term projections**

Specifically, your prospective investors should see financial projections for the first year of operations, broken down into monthly projections.

You should also provide a three-year financial projection that's broken down into yearly projections and a five-year financial projection.

TIP: It's advisable, however, to keep your five-year projection separate from your business plan, but readily available in case a potential investor asks to see it.

When you project business growth, be sure to consider the current state of your market, trends in labour and costs, and the possibility of needing additional funding for future expansion.

3. Make sure start-up fees are accounted for

Never forget to include fees for permits, licenses, and equipment in your short-term projections.

You should also keep the difference between variable and fixed costs in mind when making your projections and differentiate between the two wherever necessary. Variable costs are usually placed under the "costs for goods sold" category.

4. Go beyond your income statement

While your income statement is the basic measuring tool by which projected expenses and revenue can be conveyed, a solid financial projection will go beyond that to include projected balance sheets that show a breakdown of your assets, liabilities, and equity, among other things.

You'd also do well to include cash flow projections that reveal cash movement through the company within a given period.

Estimates of the amount you plan on borrowing as well as expected interest payments on those loans should also be included.

Furthermore, you should make sure your financial projections are all in accordance to the GAAP.
TIP: If you're new to financial reporting or don't understand the last paragraph, then you may want to consider hiring an accountant to review your projections.

5. **Offer two scenarios only**

Although you need to go beyond the simple income statement, remember that where financial projections are concerned, potential investors really want to see only two scenarios: The best- and worst-case scenarios. Anything more than those two are superfluous and may just cause unnecessary confusion, so skip it.

Finally...

To sum up, this section should tell potential investors how much money you need now and in the near future, your preferred type of funding and terms, and how you intend to use the funds.

NOTE: Take note that the intended use of the funds is a vital piece of information for potential investors and would-be creditors, which is why you need to explain it in this section.

It's also important to include all pertinent business-related information that can possibly affect the future financial situation of your company. A trend analysis for your financial statements is also very helpful, especially if you present it with graphs, as this is easier to see.

TIP: Above all, you should strive to make reasonable and clear assumptions. As previously mentioned, financial forecasting is both a science and an art. You'll need to make several assumptions, but you'll also have to be realistic when making those assumptions. Going overboard will likely raise red flags for potential investors, so always make sure your projections are backed up by solid research.

Calculating Your Start-up Costs

What are start-up costs?

These are the expenses you have to deal with before your new nail salon business can actually begin operations and earn revenue.

The concept of start-up costs is very important in tax law because these costs are not considered as deductible expenses, unlike most of the other business costs. You will, instead, need to amortize these costs over the course of a few months or years.

This means you'll only be able to deduct part of the start-up costs each year.

And you can only determine and take full deduction on your other expenses after you have determined start-up costs.

The first step

The first step in calculating the start-up costs of your business is to gather all of the expense receipts from business-related transactions.

Next, determine the exact date when your nail salon business opened and then separate the receipts into two piles: one pile for the expenses from before your business opened and another pile for expenses incurred after the opening day.

The next step is to remove all of the receipts for items such as research costs, taxes, and deductible interest from the pile receipts before opening day.
These costs can immediately be deducted.

Finally, add together all the remaining receipts belonging to your "before opening date" pile. The sum is your total start-up costs, which have to be amortized.

Amortization is usually set over a period of 18 months, and expenses like hiring and training costs, pre-opening advertising, and travel expenses to meet potential suppliers are usually included in the amortized start-up costs.

How to Obtain Business Grants

When starting a business there can be some huge barriers standing in your way, among the biggest of which are start-up costs and other business-related expenses.

You may be planning to take out a loan for the purpose of starting your nail salon business.

Why don't you consider applying for grants from the government or from private organizations instead?

There are several reasons why grants are better than a loan, the most obvious of which is the fact that grants don't need to be repaid.

How exactly can you obtain a business grant and turn your simple idea into a thriving nail salon business?

Read on to find out. The Catalog of Federal Domestic Assistance is a good place for you to search for a specific grant you can apply for because it contains a list of all grants available for small nail salon businesses.

The catalog also indicates what type of business qualifies for a particular grant, so you can immediately determine which grants your nail salon business is likely to qualify for.

Another option is for you to visit the Small Business Administration's website, which promotes federal grant programs that offer almost $2 billion to small businesses, particularly those focusing on providing technological solutions to existing business issues.

Once you have identified the grant programs you will be applying for, you should start preparing a business plan.

Take note that grant organizations base their approval or rejection of your application on the contents of your nail salon business plan.

- Your plan should therefore include a statement of purpose that is clearly written and effectively defines the goals of your company.

- A good nail salon business description, an outline of your short-term and long-term goals, a discussion on planned marketing strategies, and a projected financial analysis should also be part of your plan.

The financial section of your plan is very important because organizations usually measure the worth of a candidate based on how you plan to use the grant money.

You should therefore make sure that your financial analysis and hypothetical budget are both conservative and realistic.

When your nail salon business plan is complete, it's time to create your actual grant proposal. If you have previous experience in creating such a proposal, then you can save some money by writing the proposal yourself.

However, if you've never written a grant proposal before, then it would be wise to hire the services of a professional writer.

Make sure your proposal includes schematics, reports, and some basic information on planned projects that are likely to be influenced by the grant funds.

Furthermore, grant reviewers are likely to appreciate such attention to detail, which may be seen as a strong commitment to your product.

In this case, the reviewers will be more likely to approve your applying for grant funds.

Complete your grant application by including an updated list of contacts.

This list should start with the contact details of the top-level employees.

It should also include the contact details of individuals who can provide important details on the supplementary materials included in your application. Make sure that all pertinent information on your nail salon business and requested files by the grant organization are included in your application.

If your application lacks any of these files, then the grant is likely to be denied or the processing could be very slow. Submit your application only when you're sure that it's complete.

It's also a good idea to have your grant application reviewed by family, friends, and colleagues so grammatical errors can be cleared up and anything you may have overlooked can be pointed out to you. And as a final review process, you should schedule a reading session together with your staff, so you can correct any identified problems.

Above all, you should be patient.

Take note that the process of getting approved for grants may take longer to complete than the process of getting approved for loans.

This is because grant applications are reviewed a number of times and most grant organizations have to go through thousands of applications at a time.

Getting Insurance for Your Nail Salon Business

So, you have an idea for a good nail salon business venture; you even have the name for your new nail salon business already.

And you've also proceeded to create a business plan and a proposal for a grant application.

What else do you need to do prior to actually operating your nail salon business?

You will need good insurance.

This is actually one of the most important steps you need to take when starting a nail salon business.

Take note that if anything happened to your business equipment, tools, and supplies, you're likely to lose a considerable amount of money if you don't take out insurance for your business right from the start. In the same way, if someone should get injured in any way inside your business premises and make a claim, you may have to shell out all of your savings taking care of legal costs and compensation unless you have adequate business insurance coverage.

Here are some of the benefits you can get from the right insurance policy:

1. Your stocks and supplies will all be covered against any damage or loss, so you can replace them without cost in case of accidents or theft.

2. The right business insurance typically covers legal expenses that may be necessary in case a client dies or gets hurt in any way within the premises of your nail salon business.

3. Having the right policy also protects you in case a client makes claims for damages as a result of a treatment that was performed in your nail salon. Take note that legal costs in such cases can really add up and you just might lose your business if you don't have insurance that covers these costs.

4. If the insurance policy you choose has goods-in-transit coverage, then you're also protected in case any of your stocks get lost or damaged while making their way to you. Since stocks typically involve a high cost, you may lose a considerable amount of money for replacement if you don't have the appropriate insurance coverage.

5. Nail salon furniture and equipment are also significantly costly, so you naturally want to keep them protected against any damage or theft. The right insurance policy will definitely offer such protection.

6. If the property where your nail salon business is housed gets damaged by such incidences as fire, your insurance policy will cover the costs.

7. Since you're likely hiring employees, then you'll likely be required to take out employer's liability insurance as well. If any of your staff members get injured or unfortunately dies in a work-related accident and family members make a claim against you, then the insurance policy should sufficiently cover the legal costs.

If you've already started setting up your very own nail salon business, then you shouldn't forget to take out the correct insurance.

Even if you're starting small or running the business from home, it's still important to get a separate insurance for your nail salon business. Your household insurance isn't likely to cover any business-related accidents. And if you do decide to operate your business from home, then you should inform your household insurance provider about it. If you don't and they find out about it, you household insurance could be rendered invalid. Insurance is even more important if your business is located on separate premises.

The good news is that there are lots of great places where you can get good advice on the different types of insurance that you may need for your new nail salon business.

An insurance agent is probably the best person for you to approach if you're looking for advice on getting insurance for your nail salon business.

More specifically, you should hire the services of an agent for an insurance company that specializes on nail salon business insurance rather than a general insurance company.

You have to understand that you'll be dealing with a totally different set of risks and challenges with a business than you would with a car or with your home.

Getting insurance from a company that specializes in nail salon business insurance assures you that the agent you're dealing with really knows what he's talking about.

You can expect the insurance agent to lay out several different insurance options for you.

These options can range from liability insurance for your nail salon business to auto insurance.

You may also be offered property insurance as well as loss of business coverage, which protects your interests in case a fire breaks out and you end up without a business to run for a month or so.

It's important for you to ask questions and make sure you understand what each type of insurance covers you for so you can be sure to make an informed decision as to which types of insurance you're going to get.

More often than not, you'll be presented with more insurance options than you can afford.

There's also a possibility that the insurance agent you're consulting will present you with more insurance options than your business actually needs.
This makes it even more important for you to understand what each type of insurance covers.

Furthermore, the start of a business is usually a time when you will have to take a few risks by taking out less insurance than your nail salon business needs.

You'll have to decide how much you can afford to spend for insurance and which type of insurance is the most needed by your nail salon business.

Once you've determined this, you can leave the other types of insurance for later.

Most nail salon businesses start only with loss of business coverage, others with liability insurance. The point is to get only the most important insurance coverage that you can afford for starters. As your company grows, it will become more important for you to protect your nail salon business' assets. And the good news is that you may able to afford it at that time.

Aside from the insurance that you have previously identified as a need for your nail salon business, there may also be other types of insurance that your customers expect you to have.

You can work on getting these additional insurance types when the right time comes.

It's definitely a good idea to compare a few insurance policies before making any commitment, since there can be a huge difference in the cost of premiums as well as in the benefits you get from the policy. The key is to check out the coverage and then choose the policy that best matches your preferences and needs.

How to Trademark Your Nail Salon Business Name and Logo

If you have just put up a new nail salon business, you should be careful not to stop at choosing a name and logo for it.

You should also make sure that the name and logo you chose is adequately protected.

This is especially important if one of your business goals is to create an instantly recognizable brand. The best way to protect your business name and logo is to have it trademarked.

Take note that a trademark is also used to protect symbols, drawings, and any other character associated with your nail salon business, much like a patent protects inventions.

The whole process of getting your business name and logo trademarked is a relatively simple one.

However, it often takes several months for your trademark registration to really become official. Following is a quick guide on how you can protect your business name and logo by getting it trademarked.

1.   Choose the name and design the logo for your new nail salon business.

     You have to make sure, of course, that the name and logo you choose are not yet being used by any other company.
     More importantly, you need to ensure that such name and logo have not already been trademarked by someone else.

You can check the database of the official trademark office to make sure you won't run into any legal problems with your chosen name and logo.

2. Once you have established that your chosen nail salon business name and logo are not yet trademarked, request for and fill-out the necessary paperwork.

   Once the paperwork has been filled out and submitted to the Patent and Trademark Office, the processing of your application for registration will officially begin.

3. Allow five months for the processing to be completed.

   If five months have passed and you still have not received any notification of your trademark having been filed, you may check on its status. Take note, though, that it usually takes between five and seven months for a trademark registration process to be completed.

4. Once you receive notification of your trademark having been filed, obtain a copy of it from the trademark office.

   Take note that you will be asked for your registration number when you make the request for a copy of your trademark certificate.

5. Between the fifth and sixth year of your trademark registration, make sure that an

"Affidavit of Use" is filed, so as to prevent other companies from using your trademarked name and logo.

You should remember to file two other affidavits as well before every 10-year period of owning the trademark has passed.

Writing an LLC
Operating Agreement

Limited Liability Corporation, or LLC, is the ideal set-up for start-up companies and small businesses because it requires the business owner to take on only limited liability for the company.

And the good news is that creating an LLC is fairly simple and inexpensive. Take note that the operations of an LLC are governed by the LLC operating agreement.

You'll therefore need to learn how to write your LLC operating agreement.

Here is a step-by-step guide:

1. Gather basic information such as the company name and location as well as the names and physical addresses of the members of your company. You should also note your agent's name.

2. Gather all financial information.

   This includes each member's initial contribution to the company and how much each of them will own in terms of percentage of company interest. You can choose to have either a single-member or multi-member LLC.

   For example, you could choose to initially make a contribution of $100 and own a hundred percent of the company.

   What's important is for all company members to be included in your LLC operating agreement.

3. Choose and download a sample agreement.

   Of course, you can choose to write your own agreement from scratch, but working from a sample would definitely make the process much easier for you.

   While operating agreements aren't really that complex, the language used can be very governmental, and basing your agreement on a sample will help ensure that the language is interpreted correctly.

4. Determine if you need the services of a registered agent.

   Take note that there's a slight difference in the LLC laws of each state.

   The operating agreement typically has a space that needs to be filled in for the registered agent. If your state's requirements allow it, you can be the one to fill in this space.

5. Check the "Business Purpose" section of your sample agreement and make sure it includes the statement that indicates your company's purpose as engaging in lawful acts or activities for which an LLC may be formed.

   You should also check the language in the "Term" section. "Indefinitely" is commonly used for the term.

   In the terms of dissolution, "by a majority" is also commonly used.

6. You should also check the language in the "Management" section.

   A majority of small nail salon businesses are managed by the members as a whole, but you also have the option of getting managers for your nail salon business, especially if there are active and passive members.

   Whatever you decide, make sure your agreement contains the appropriate language as to how your company will operate.

7. Personalize the sample agreement by inserting the data from the notes you took as per Step 1 and Step 2. Be sure to include the necessary signature lines.

8. Print the agreement as well as a list of all members with their respective addresses and then staple them together.

   Let all members sign the agreement, have it photocopied, and then provide each member with a copy.

   Be sure to keep the original somewhere safe and have additional copies in your files for reference.

Take note that this step-by-step guide does not constitute legal advice.

If there's anything about forming an LLC that you don't understand, it's still best to seek the advice of an attorney.

Writing a Company Brochure

A company brochure, also known as a corporate brochure, is an excellent way of introducing your nail salon business to your target market.

That is, of course, if you do it right.

The very first things you need to take into consideration are the logo, font, and color you use on your brochure.

People will only learn about your nail salon business if they read the brochure, and they are more likely to read a brochure if the cover has an attractive design, which is why your choice of logo, font, and color is very important.

Take note as well that people are more likely to patronize your nail salon business if you're able to build a connection with them and if you're able to establish in their minds the thought that you can be trusted.

The best way to do this using a brochure is to include pertinent information such as the background and history of your company, what you have to offer, and how you intend to deliver whatever it is you're offering. You may also include information on how your company intends to serve the community as a whole.

Furthermore, you'll need to provide an explanation of what the brochure itself is all about.

- Is it just about the organization or does it present the products and services as well?

- Is it all about the industry and what role your company plays in its development?

- Is it for a specific event where your company is a participant or is it a detailed brochure of your company?

And of course, you'll have to tell the reader at the outset what the brochure's relevance to him is.

Therefore, before you even start writing your company brochure, you'll first have to think about what you want the brochure to portray and who your target audience is.

You may want to set-up a brainstorming session with your company's key personnel for this purpose.

And take note that even as your brochure contains all the necessary information as discussed above, it should remain concise and easy to read.

You should also make it easy for the reader to select which particular piece of information he wants to read. This can be achieved through the use of headings and sub-titles.

As long as you keep these tips in mind, you should be able to create a company brochure that truly presents your nail salon business in a positive light.

Leasing Space

Having enough space for your business is one of the most critical factors in operating your new business. In choosing retail sales space, you'll have to take several things into consideration.

Among these things are good visibility of the location from the street, and easy access for your customers. You'll also have to decide if you're going to build, buy, or rent your retail sales space.

There are many advantages to renting space as opposed to buying or building.

Maintenance, flexibility, and taxes are perhaps the three most important advantages.

Maintenance

If you rent retail sales space, you'll be responsible only for a bit of routine maintenance issues like the replacement of light bulbs, repairing uninsured damages caused by negligence on your part, and cleaning the premises.

The good news for you is that major maintenance issues like electrical, plumbing, air conditioning, heating, and structural problems are the responsibility of your landlord.

This means that if your roof starts to leak, it will be your landlord's responsibility to have it repaired.

Knowing that your rent already covers major maintenance issues makes it so much easier for you to budget your company's available funds.

Flexibility

Renting space helps you avoid being forced to stay at the same location even when it's no longer practical to do so.

Even if you have a lease contract for a specific period, that's still a lot better than getting locked into a commercial mortgage.

If the demographics in your area change, then it will be much easier to relocate your nail salon business if you're simply leasing or renting space.

This also holds true for the time when your nail salon business has grown such that you need more space. Furthermore, you won't have to worry about selling your existing location if you have to move to a new place, which is an issue you'll have to deal with if you own the space.

Taxes

It's very easy to understand the advantages of renting space where taxes are concerned.

Rental payments are considered business expenses and are therefore deductible.

On the other hand, only the interest that you pay for commercial mortgages is deductible.

You have to consider as well, the fact that commercial property often doesn't appreciate as much as residential properties, which means your property may accrue very little equity over time.

When you weight this against the 100% deductibility of commercial rent, you'll realize how advantageous it is to simply lease retail space.

Now that you understand the benefits of leasing retail sales space, you'll have to learn how to find the perfect location for your nail salon business.

Remember that leasing will affect not only your company's profit, but also its ability to grow as well as the satisfaction level of your employees.

So, before you go out looking for space to rent, you'll have to know exactly what you are looking for.

Here's how to identify the perfect retail sales space for your nail salon business:

1. Determine how much space your nail salon business needs now and how much it may need in the future. The rule of thumb in determining space requirements is to have 175-250 sq. ft. of space for each person who will be working at the location.

2. Contact a real estate agent and seek advice in finding a suitable commercial space.

   Agents typically have the inside scoop on what'd going on in the real estate market and they can advise you properly on which particular properties are ideal for your purposes.
   It's a good idea to contact a real estate firm that specializes in office space rentals.

3. Discuss any necessary improvements with your potential landlord.

   Take note that improvements are usually subject to serious negotiations, especially if there are lots of vacancies.

   You would also do well to check out the parking space.

   Does the rental offer a number of slots you can set aside for yourself and your employees, or would you have to compete with the public for street parking?

4. You may be able to reduce rental cost by either sharing space or looking out for incubators.

   You could share your reception area, rest rooms, and conference rooms with another small firm to reduce your rental costs – that is, if you're okay with having less privacy.

   Incubators are small unused areas in a larger building which are usually offered for lease at much lower costs.

   These are also good options for a small nail salon business like yours, provided it meets with your requirements, of course.

5. You may also want to consider renting an all-inclusive suite.

The rate for executive office suites is usually higher, but they usually come fully-furnished and provide you with access to meeting rooms and office equipment, thus significantly reducing your up-front costs.

Many of these suites even come with a receptionist.

6. Before signing a lease contract, be sure to review it exhaustively.

   Check the indicated monthly payment, how long the lease is for, what maintenance and repair concerns the landlord will be responsible for, and things like annual rent increases in accordance with inflation.

   You'd also do well to check if there are provisions concerning the possibility of terminating the lease early as well as provisions regarding internet connections, cable service, telephone lines, and other company needs.

   Other important details for you to review include the date of occupancy, right of refusal for the adjoining space, security, and other amenities.

7. Finally, it's a good idea for you to hire a qualified real estate attorney.

   Make sure the attorney specializes in negotiations for leases and that he knows your area.
   It's a bonus if he has dealt with the same kind of nail salon business in the past.

This is important because lease negotiations typically cover hundreds of terms, which makes it a definite advantage to have someone who's gone through it all before on your side.

Managing Your Employees

Once you have your new nail salon business in place, you'll have to deal with managing your employees, which can be a very tricky process.

If you're not careful, you just might end up babysitting rather than running a successful nail salon business venture.

This is especially true if a majority of your employees are paid very low hourly rates.

You're lucky if you can hire wonderful employees who don't give you any problems.

However, you'll still have to find effective ways of keeping these wonderful employees in your nail salon business, and that's where good employee management comes in.

Perhaps the most important aspect of employee management is your ability to set very clear goals and communicate your company objectives very clearly to your employees.

Take note that goal-setting and communicating objectives have to be done regularly.

The more you communicate with your employees in an honest and open manner, the easier it will be for you to manage them. It's advisable to set monthly, quarterly, and annual goals. And you have to make sure the goals you set are mutual.

This means you should not be forcing your employees to work towards your own goals.

The employees themselves have to believe in those goals and they'll have to be taught how to adjust in case circumstances that keep them from attaining those goals suddenly arise.

Furthermore, you need to realize that goals don't really mean much unless employees' compensations are largely tied up with those goals.

The compensation may be in the form of bonuses, commissions, or salary percentages.

What's important is for the employees to have a good motivation for working towards the company's goals. It's also a good idea to hold a yearly meeting with all of your employees where an annual review will be conducted. During this review, you should commend your employees for the things they're doing right and discuss solutions for the things that didn't quite work out.

Identifying areas of improvement and finding solutions together can give employees the assurance that they really are part of the company and that they're being valued as individuals, not just as paid workers.

Finally, another very important part of employee management is getting feedback on how YOU are doing at your job.

- How are you as a manager?

- What are you doing right?

- What else can you do to become a better manager?

You have to realize that getting feedback from your employees isn't a waste of your time.

Quite the contrary, in fact.

More often than not, the best ideas for improving a nail salon business come from the front-liners, as they're usually the ones who know exactly what the customers want.

How to Market Your
Nail Salon Business

Marketing your new nail salon business probably ranks among the most challenging aspects of putting up a business venture, not to mention that it can also be the most fun.

You should, in fact, be excited about marketing your nail salon business.

- The main purpose of marketing a nail salon business is to let your target customers know that you exist and that you have a lot of benefits to offer them.

And take note that the kind of message you convey to your target market is crucial when you market a new nail salon business.

Even if you're selling exactly the same item as your closest competitor, you're more likely to come out on top of the competition if you're able to come up with better marketing strategies and if you can successfully create a brand for your company.

Creating a brand for your company will make your nail salon business more valuable to potential customers. Regardless of what type of business you're into branding is still important.

In fact, the more you create an attractive personality around your company brand, the more you set yourself apart from the competition, thus giving your nail salon business a much better opportunity for growth.

How do you know your brand is effective?

Simple.

Market it to yourself.

Imagine that you're a would-be customer taking stock of a new player in the industry.

- Does the company brand look, sound, and feel authentic?

- Is it a fun and attractive brand?

Remember that marketing your nail salon business has to be fun, so don't take it too seriously.

And even while you're working hard to create a brand, you should always remain true to yourself.

That is what will make your brand truly authentic. And an authentic brand is something your competition can never take away.

Using business cards to market your salon

As a nail salon owner, you probably already know it's important to have business cards as part of your overall marketing and advertising strategy.

In fact, handing out business cards should be a regular endeavour to make sure you get a steady stream of clients into your nail salon business.

But, do know how you can best use these business cards to your advantage?

What should you print on your cards to make them effective marketing tools?

To start with, a business card can be your best business marketing tool as long as you know how to use it. It can easily be distributed and people you give it to are more likely to pass it on to others than they would a leaflet or brochure.

A business card can travel miles without you even knowing it!

Effective use of business cards to market your nail salon involves massive and regular distribution. You could perhaps aim to distribute at least ten business cards each day, or even more if possible.

On average, people get three clients for every ten business cards distributed. Therefore, the more cards you hand out, the more new clients you're likely to get. Of course, you can't just distribute your business cards anywhere and expect to get the attention of your target market. Be sure to distribute them at strategic locations frequented by your prospective customers. Since you're running a nail salon, you're likely aiming to catch the interest of adult women or maybe even the growing number of appearance-conscious professional men. It's therefore a good idea to distribute your business cards outside supermarkets and hairdressers as well as within the busy downtown area usually traversed by young professionals. If possible, spend a few seconds chatting with a prospect as you give them your card.

Three versions

It's also advisable for you to have three different versions of your business card printed.

1. An appointment card is a business card with an appointment time indicated at the back.

2. A referral card is a business card indicating a referral system you may be offering.

3. Finally, a new prospects card is a business card that describes the services you offer.

Regardless of what type of business card you distribute, though, make sure it indicates what you specialise in. For example, there could be a line on the back that says, "The best French tips in the county!" This immediately informs a potential client what you generally do in your nail salon.

While a business card only covers a small aspect of your overall marketing and advertising campaign, it can be a vital part of your strategy.

In fact, it may be one of your most valuable marketing tools, which is why you need to learn how to use it the right way.

An essential part of ensuring the success of any business is learning how to maximise your resources.

Therefore, you shouldn't waste even a single business card. Use it properly as a marketing tool and you'll surely enjoy the long-term results as you see your nail salon business becoming more and more successful.

Finally…

Here are some final useful tips on how to ensure the success of your nail salon business:

1. Prepare Everything

The most important part of setting up any business venture is the planning stage. If you plan all your moves carefully, everything else you need to do can be very easily accomplished.

This is why writing a business plan is the necessary first step in setting up your nails salon business.

Your business plan should describe the services you plan to offer, the hours of operation you plan to have, the fees and charges for each type of service, the equipment and tools you'll need for the business, your target location, your target market, and how much you expect to spend on start-up costs.

You should also include your financial projections and marketing plan.

2. Make Detailed Cost Estimations

Needless to say, the cost of setting up the business is one of the most important considerations.

When you make your cost estimations, be sure not to leave out even the tiniest expense.

The estimation should cover not just property rental and equipment cost, but also the salaries of your employees for the first year of operation and the materials you'll be using down to the last cotton ball.

3. Consider Applying for Grants

Most people who start a business don't really have enough saved up to cover start-up costs and the operational costs for the first few months of the business.

Remember that it'll take time to build a client base, so you'll need enough money to cover your first few months in the business. You may want to apply for grants, which can definitely help you manage your expenses and operational costs. Your cost estimates will guide you in deciding how much to apply for when you start searching for the perfect grant.

4. Learn as Much as You Can about the Business

Read up on nail art-related magazines, newspaper articles, and journals. Check out websites of nail artists and technicians as well as other things that offer valuable information about the business of running a nail salon and how to go about setting it up.

5. Find Out What the Experts Have to Say

Take your cue from nail care professionals who've gone down the same road before you. Read blogs by nail salon experts and ask any nail care professional you know what they think are the most important things a nail salon owner should take care of. You should also ask them what you need to avoid doing so as not to compromise your business. It's best to get advice from those whose nail salon businesses won't be in competition with yours, of course.

Simply by following the tips above, you should be able to look forward to a flourishing nails salon business of your own.

Good luck.

Made in United States
Troutdale, OR
01/30/2024